POUCH PORTIONS

A Bariatric Survival Guide & Recipe Book

By Mandy Towle

Contents

ACKNOWLEDGEMENTS

I dedicate this book to my husband Martin. Without all of his love and belief in me I couldn't have made it through. He is my rock when I feel it's all too much and my conscience when I stray from the path.

 I'd also like to thank my wonderful family and friends who've supported me in my journey, and of course special thanks to my Consultant, Mr M Riera MD, FRCS Ed (Gen Surg) and his wonderful Bariatric Team, Bryony, Hailey and Viv, to name a few, who are always there to help and without whom none of this would have been possible.

PREFACE

So dear PP reader,

You've probably bought this book because you're thinking about having bariatric surgery, or you're just setting out on your new post bariatric life.

If you're looking for some insider info on what to expect after your surgery you've come to the right place.

Throughout this book I'll tell you about my experiences as well as give you some of my favourite PP bariatric recipes, useful food plans and helpful tools.

I really hope you enjoy this book as much as you do your new life.

I just know it's going to be amazing!

IMPORTANT DISCLAIMER

I don't profess to be medically trained or a dietician and you should ALWAYS follow the advice given to you by your own Bariatric Team as they know your case individually and what
is right for you.

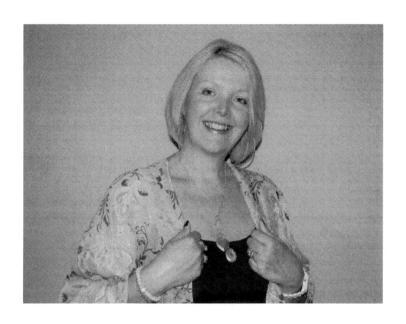

About Me

Welcome dear Pouch Portions, (PP) reader,

Here's a little bit about me - I'll try not to bore you too much.

At 50, after many years of struggling with my weight and trying every diet plan on the planet I decided my only solution if I wanted to live to see my 70th birthday was to have bariatric surgery.

Now I know that sounds melodramatic, but at 22.5 stones, (315 lbs.) my health was deteriorating rapidly.

I had high blood pressure, extreme joint pain, breathlessness, early NAFLD, (non-alcoholic fatty liver disease), and badly swollen feet and ankles making mobility increasingly difficult.

I had to do something about it if I wanted to see my grandchildren grow up.

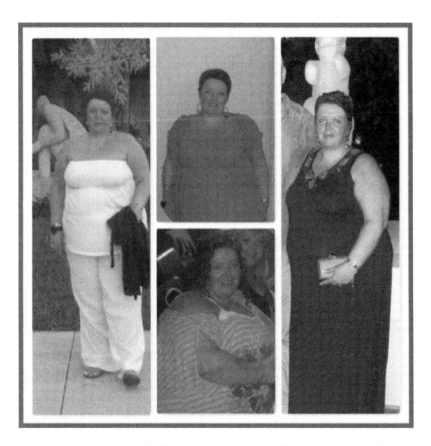

Pictures of me before my op at my heaviest weight

12 months later in May 2016, I had my Roux-en-Y gastric bypass, and I can honestly say it was the best decision I ever made.

My only regret is that I didn't do it sooner.
My life has changed dramatically for the better since
my surgery. I've already lost 7.5 stones, (105 lbs.) and
I'm not even a year post op.

I don't need the medication for my high blood
pressure as it's now normal, my mobility is 100%
better and I don't get breathless or have joint pain from
walking or climbing the stairs. My feet and ankles are
no longer swollen - I can actually wear regular sizes in
shoes and boots which is the best feeling ever.

And I don't have to shop at the overpriced "fat shops"
any more as I've gone from a size 26 to a size 16.

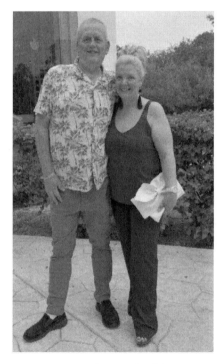

Me now with my hubby, Martin

I could go on and on as the list of positives is endless, (but I won't).

Post bariatric life is good dear PP reader and I wish you good luck with yours.

Mandy

Now onto the reason you got this book...

So You Want Bariatric Surgery?

Weight loss surgery is NOT the "easy option "and if that's what you think then think again!

A lot of people think it's going to be like waving a magic wand – they'll have the op and their fat will vanish overnight.

That would be great, but in reality the surgery is only a weight loss tool. There's still an awful lot of hard work involved afterwards like changes to your diet, activity levels and lifestyle before you to reach your perfect weight.

To have weight loss surgery on the NHS, NICE guidelines say:

- You must have a BMI of 40 or more, or between 35 and 40 with other significant illnesses that would improve if you lost weight e.g. type 2 diabetes or high blood pressure.
- You must have tried all non-surgical options but haven't achieved or maintained beneficial weight loss
- You must be fit for anaesthesia and surgery.
- You must commit to long-term follow-up.

If you think that you meet the criteria and you are positive that it's what you want, the next step is to ask your GP to refer you to the bariatric team.

Then your own bariatric journey can begin!

How to follow the Liver Shrinkage Diet without cheating!

So you've got your weight loss surgery date. That's absolutely fantastic!

I know that I was so excited when I got mine I could have cried!

But now you need to start thinking seriously about doing the Liver Shrinkage Diet, (or LSD for short). Different bariatric teams recommend different LSD's, but in a nutshell it's a very low calorie diet that will shrink your liver so that the bariatric surgeon can do his stuff.

If you have an enlarged or fatty liver, as lots of us "curvy" folk do, it makes it really difficult, sometimes nigh on impossible, to carry out the surgery as your liver has to be lifted up out of the way so the surgeon can get to your stomach.

If it's too big they will cancel your operation and we definitely don't want that do we!

Telford & Shropshire CCG who did my gastric bypass insist on a minimum 2 weeks LSD before the operation, and I had a choice of the following options:

- A very low calorie liquid diet like Slim-fast 4 times a day, (I used Exante shakes for my LSD as they have a wide range of flavours so I didn't get bored), plus 1-2 litres of calorie free fluid like water or no added sugar squash.

- 4 tins of low calorie soup like weight watchers and 4 low fat yoghurts like Muller Light, plus 1 pint of semi-skimmed milk.

- A small bowl of plain cereal or 1 medium slice of toast with a scraping of butter for breakfast. 1 slice of bread or 2 crisp breads with salad, (no dressing) plus a small portion of fish, cheese, eggs or baked beans for lunch. Then for dinner, 1 small potato or 2 tablespoons of pasta or rice with any leafy green vegetables, (you can have sweet corn, carrots, peas and beetroot but they contain more starch so you can only have 1 tablespoon) and one small portion of either meat, fish, cheese, eggs, quorn, or tofu. On top of all this you can have as much water, tea, coffee, low calorie squash and low calorie fizzy drinks as you like, but you have to limit fruit juice to one small glass, (100ml) per day. If you are diabetic your LSD will be different as the normal LSD will lower your blood glucose levels, so you'll need to chat to your Diabetic nurse or GP to see what they recommend. And as well as following your bariatric team's LSD's you must take a multivitamin once a day. It can be any complete multivitamin, (I used Aldi's own brand but you can use whatever brand you like. I'm not endorsing Aldi!). It prepares your body for your operation, and it also gets you into good habits of taking vitamins daily – after surgery you'll be taking them for the rest of your life!

You will probably have a few side effects while on your LSD, mainly constipation because of the reduced fibre in your diet.

To help prevent it you should drink plenty, 2 to 3 litres a day. And if that doesn't work ask your doctor for some Fybogel and take 1 to 2 sachets a day.

The other problem will be that your body goes into Ketosis, which is when your body burns fat instead of carbohydrates. This causes bad breath, (my other half moaned about my bad breath constantly!) headaches, mild dizziness and nausea. Sounds unpleasant, but chewing gum, drinking plenty and having sugar free mints helps.

If you are serious about having the surgery none of this will matter. All I was interested in was shrinking my liver so my operation didn't get cancelled!

My tips to get you through your LSD are:

- Try out your LSD for a few days before you actually need to start it proper. This helps you plan how you'll cope when you have to do it for real!

- Be mindful of what you are eating. Eat slowly. Savour it and taste every mouthful.

- If it's killing you and you really, really, really need to eat something extra snack on cucumber and cherry tomatoes to keep you going.

- Stay as busy as you can – you tend to think constantly about food when you're bored. Do something you enjoy to take your mind off it. I love to paint and make cards so that's what I did, (I made enough cards to last me the year!).

- Let everyone know you're on your LSD and that you'll probably be tired and irritable.

- And if all else fails, have some early nights – the extra beauty sleep will do you good.

And remember it's only 2 weeks to prepare yourself for your new life!

Before Your Weight Loss Surgery

Bariatric teams all work slightly differently, but I thought I'd tell you about my great experience with Telford & Shrewsbury CCG.

After referral by my GP back in February 2015, my first appointment letter dropped through my letter box and in April 2015 I went to the Princess Royal Hospital in Telford with my other half.

Before I saw my Consultant, I had my height and weight taken. Next I went in to see Mr Riera who went through my medical history with me. As my BMI was over 50 and I suffered from high blood pressure I was a perfect candidate. He explained the procedures available; the gastric bypass, the sleeve, the band etc. and asked if I had a preference? You are involved in making choices every step of the way.

Of course I'd investigated it loads and I knew that I wanted the Roux-en-Y Gastric Bypass as it is the gold standard weight loss surgery. I really didn't feel confident about having the sleeve as it is a relatively new procedure – although I do know quite a few people who have had it and done really well on it.

He agreed and said that my next appointment would be an educational one with the Bariatric nurse. It was a half day group induction about the process, procedures and what to expect. And that was that really. I wasn't there long. We came away feeling very positive.

My educational appointment was on August the 3rd 2015, 4 months after my first appointment. Again it was at the Princess Royal Hospital Telford in the Education Centre and there were around 20 people and almost everyone had come with their support partners – it was great to see.

The Bariatric Nurse Specialist, Sister Bryony Price, gave a great session explaining the types of surgery and the benefits and risks involved, what to expect while in hospital including medications and wound care, driving after the op and exercise.

My other half asked loads of questions. I was really glad he was there with me as he asked things I hadn't even thought of.

This was followed by a session on the "Liver Shrinkage Diet" (LSD), "eating after surgery", "nutritional drinks and supplements after surgery", "troubleshooting problems with eating", "multivitamins" and "lifelong eating".

We all had a quick coffee break followed by a session on "Mindful Eating to prepare for weight loss surgery and beyond" and how to create a "Relapse Recovery Plan" by the Mental Health Eating Disorders Specialist Dietician, Vivienne Love. I found this particularly interesting as I'd been reading up on mindfulness and meditation, and my other half really enjoyed the food craving section.

All in all it was a really good training session and we both came away with lots of information about what to expect and how to cope. I don't know if your bariatric team offers this type of thing, but they really should as it was a brilliant morning!

My next appointment was with the Mental Health Eating Disorders Specialist Dietician who I'd met at the educational appointment.

I was a bit apprehensive about it beforehand, but I needn't have worried. She was great and I told her about the on-line mindfulness course I'd started, my morning meditation and I showed her my LSD plan. She seemed very impressed and she was the one who suggested I write about my journey.

(Thank you Viv x)

Anyway, everything must have been ok with my mental health, (although my other half would beg to differ!) because on the 18th of December 2015 I was back in Mr Riera's consulting room where he gave me a surgery date of the 14th of March 2016, and told me to pop along to Pre-Op for my assessment!

I was ecstatic!

We were then taken to Pre-Op Assessment where I had my blood pressure taken, height, weight, sats, (oxygen saturation) MRSA nose swab, bloods and ECG.
The Pre -Op Sister asked me a series of health related questions which she filled in on her computer and at the end it gave a "suitability for surgery" rating of Red – not suitable, Amber – Possible and Green – good to go.

Mine was green so I was fine. Then she gave me a couple of Ranitidine tablets to take the evening before and the morning of my op, (because I suffered from acid reflux) and told me I would get confirmation of my date in the post.

I received my letter on the 18th of February 2016 which was about 4 weeks before my surgery date. This gave me plenty of time to do my LSD for the 2 weeks prior to my op.

Unfortunately, I work in a GP surgery where germs and viruses are rife, and a few days before my op I started to develop a cough. I tried to ignore it and be as positive as I could.

"Positivity" is my mantra.
It was just a cough. It would go away.

But it got worse!

I carried on with my LSD as if I was having the surgery. I was determined I was going to have the op. On the eve of my op I talked long and hard with my other half and we came to the conclusion that it would probably be cancelled.

Next morning my cough didn't seem quite as bad, but maybe that was wishful thinking. Positivity and all that!

We arrived at the Royal Shrewsbury Hospital at about 7 am – I'd starved from 10 the night before and had only had sips of water after so was dying of thirst, especially with the cough!

I was shown to a room where I put on a theatre gown, PJ bottoms, slippers and my dressing gown.
The anaesthetist came to see me and asked if I was fit and well. I told him about my cough, (which at the time was being particularly quiet!) and he assured me it would be fine.

Then Mr Riera came in and asked the anaesthetist if I was ok for surgery and he said yes! My other half and I looked at each other; was this really happening!

We were shown into another room and the hospital was so hot and stuffy that my tickly cough started to get worse, especially as I couldn't have a drink to ease it. I started to use my inhaler to try and make it stop.

But then the Admissions Sister started to complete my paperwork and take my vitals. My SATs, (oxygen saturation) were low and my temperature was high!

"I'm not happy with these readings Mandy", she frowned "something's not quite right".

She listened to my chest and said she could hear something – I already knew she was right as it had felt uncomfortable since that morning.

Anyway, to cut a long story short, Mr Riera, my consultant called me back to the consulting room and said he thought we should leave it for today and I totally agreed as by now I was feeling awful and had had enough.

Obviously I was very disappointed, but I didn't want to have the op and then end up being really poorly. A cough and stitches are a bad combo me thinks?!

So we went home, and it was a good job we did.

It turned out I had a really bad chest infection and was off work for over a week!

I did get a date for a couple of months later folks, and now I'm 34 weeks post op.

"Never Give Up!"

Your Gastric Bypass – What To Expect

So my new date came through – May the 16th 2016.

To avoid the previous disaster with the "chest infection episode" I took the week off work prior to my op, (I'm very lucky that my boss is so understanding).

I'd done my LSD for 2 weeks beforehand, taken my Ranitidine tablets and fasted the night before. I felt fit as a fiddle, but I took a couple of Paracetamol with my usual medications that morning just to be sure my temperature was ok.

I went to Hospital for 7:30am with my other half in tow and saw the anaesthetist, signed the consent form with my Consultant, and had all the checks done by the Sister. As it had been a while I had to have a repeat MRSA nose swab, bloods, sats, blood pressure, urine, temperature and weight and guess what?

 I'd lost 10kg since March! Bonus!

All of my results were fine, so needless to say I was as happy as Larry.

Then I kissed my other half and walked down to theatre with the porter. Strangely, I didn't feel a bit nervous? I'd waited such a long time for this day to finally arrive!

I was greeted by the anaesthetist and theatre team who got me to lie on the operating table, all the time chatting to me, telling me exactly what was going on and putting me at ease.

Someone put me on a blood pressure monitor, ECG machine and sats monitor and the anaesthetist put a cannula, (a thin tube inserted into a vein to administer medication) into the back of my left hand as I'm right handed.

"I'm just going to give you something to help you relax through this face mask Mandy, ok?" he said and I nodded and looked up at the huge round theatre light above me.

The next thing I knew I was waking up on the recovery ward!

The gastric bypass took one and a half hours and I vaguely recall my consultant at my bedside saying that the operation had gone extremely well – I'd been given a dose of morphine and kept drifting in and out of sleep.

When I was more awake my Recovery Nurse showed me the morphine pump I was attached to and how to press the little green button if I felt pain.

"Don't worry", she smiled "it will only give you a small dose so there's no chance of overdose".

I pressed that green button whenever I could to keep the pain relief topped up. I couldn't see the point in being in unnecessary pain at this point – I'd advise you to do the same!

The nurse checked on me quite often and always asked what my pain was on a scale of 1 to 10 with 10 being the most.

To be honest it was always around 2 because I was so out of it. She also kept me updated about my bed availability, but it was 3 hours before one became free. I asked her if they could contact my other half as he'd be really worried as it was so long since my op – which he was. Very worried!

Then they wheeled me to the ward. I was in a lovely 4 bedded female bay with its own bathroom. The nursing staff on the ward were all fantastic. They got me into my nightie and made me comfortable.

I was on oxygen, attached to a drip of fluids to stop me becoming dehydrated as well as the morphine pump.

It's a bit awkward at first, but you soon get used to being hooked up and the incessant beeping of the alarm if you raise your hand up too high.

After my other half had been and gone I needed the toilet as my bladder was fit to burst. An HCA helped me out of bed and to the loo.

(Tip: to be allowed home you need to have passed urine)

It was difficult the first time.

You are attached to a drip and pump on wheels, you still feel unsteady on your feet, and that toilet seems far too low down! But you do manage and every time after just gets easier and easier.

I checked my wounds the first chance I got; there were just five small dressings and I couldn't really see much.

The nursing staff did my observations every hour or so, (just when I'd nodded off it seemed) so I didn't get much sleep that first night at all.

My stay was only supposed to be 2 days, but unfortunately the day after my surgery I started to feel really, really sick. I think this was because I'd stopped using the morphine pump as I didn't feel I needed it any more, (you can't go home on morphine can you!).

My consultant came to see me and said I'd better stay another night and prescribed some anti-sickness medication which the nurse gave me via my drip.

I got really tearful. I felt absolutely awful and desperately wanted to go home. I honestly began to wonder if I'd done the right thing in having the surgery because I felt so ill!

The nurse, bless her, pulled the curtains round me to give me some privacy, and my other half was allowed to visit early. I was so upset.

But the anti-sickness medication did the trick and except for one observation check during the night, I had a great night's sleep.

Next day I felt much better.

I was up and down to the toilet on my own, sitting in the chair, drinking plenty and, " Grossness Alert" I'd even opened my bowels.

(Tip: this is the second thing you need to have done before they'll discharge you)

Speaking of drinking plenty, you're expected to drink at least 3 jugs of water a day. This is difficult as you can only take tiny sips, but you really must try. You don't want to become dehydrated.

(Tip: this is the third thing you must do before being allowed home)

The consultant came to see me again and said I could go home as I was feeling ok. Yippee!

Then the Dietician came and spoke to me about what I should be doing food wise for the next six weeks, and gave me some Ensure Plus Advance drinks to have while I was recovering, as well as a bag full of medication to take home.

This is what I had, but yours may differ:

- Tinzaparin Injections, two per day for the next 20 days to prevent blood clots, (the nurse will show you how to inject yourself in your tummy before you go home. Don't worry – you get used to it).
- Paracetamol Oral Suspension, four 5ml spoonfuls each day as needed for pain.
- Lansoprazole Orodispersible tablets, one a day dissolved under your tongue.
- Dalivit Drops, liquid vitamins, 14 drops per day

(Tip: On the topic of medication, not all staff on wards may be aware of the needs of bariatric patients and I was offered tablets more than once. You must say that you can only have liquid medication or dissolvable, and if you're given effervescent Paracetamol, leave it to go flat before you take it)

I also had to take my normal blood pressure medication and water tablets until I'd seen my GP in a few weeks' time.

I was told to remove my dressings on the 4th day, have showers not baths as the stitches were dissolvable, and trim off any stitches with nail clippers close to the skin if they were poking out.

I was given a discharge letter with all of my operation details and medication instructions on, (a copy was sent to my GP) then my other half came to take me home.

(Tip: make sure you have something loose to go home in. I'd taken linen trousers but they were so uncomfortable around my tummy that I had to put my PJ bottoms back on)

I was so relieved to be discharged.

In the famous words of Dorothy from the Wizard of Oz, "There's no place like home".

The First Week After Gastric Bypass

After your op you expect to feel quite sore around your tummy area, but the worst pain I had was from trapped wind, and let me tell you, it was really painful!

During your op they pump you full of air so that they can get to all of your plumbing, and a lot of it gets trapped.

The best way to get rid of it? Keep moving.

When you stand up and walk around the wind travels down your body and out the usual way. But if you lie around in bed or on the sofa it can't escape and the pain is awful. My advice – walk around as much as you can!

I also couldn't manage the stairs to bed, even with my other half's help. I slept on my sofa for 5 days!
Just keep trying. You'll get up them eventually.

But the main problem I found was that everything took such a long time!

Each day it seemed like all I was doing was taking my medication, injecting myself, (which I had to psych myself up to do by the way) and trying my best to cram in my 6 small liquid meals and 3 pints of fluid.

Because you can only sip (don't forget that your new stomach is the size of an eggcup), it takes a lifetime to drink your meals and fluids.

And it's all very tiring after the surgery as your body is busy repairing itself. I had a few naps throughout the day and I'd still be ready for bed at 10pm. Before the surgery I never went to bed before midnight!

I also became very tearful and very emotional, crying at nothing and shouting at my other half for no reason (even though he was golden).

But having gone through that stage and safely out the other side, my advice to you would be to give yourself a break!

You've just had major surgery, be it keyhole or not, and you have permission to be weepy and emotional. It's normal and it will pass. Don't bottle it up or try to hide it. Just let it run its course.

At some point you need to get your dressings off.

I was supposed to take mine off in the shower after 4 days, (you may have a different time-scale for removing them) but as I struggled with the stairs it was five days, and boy did it make a difference!

Those pesky little wounds, with their dissolvable stitches poking out, had stuck to the plasters and did not want to come off!

I had to stay in the shower for ages until they finally came loose. I was in there so long that the water ran cold and I still had one that refused to budge. Stupidly I tugged it loose.

Big mistake!

The dressing came off, but a lot of my surrounding skin came with it. Luckily for me the wound stayed closed but it was terribly sore I can tell you!

Had I thought about it properly I should have just soaked them off in the kitchen on the fourth day.

Your New Bariatric Food Plan

After your op it's very important to follow the food plan given to you by your bariatric team.
I was given my post bariatric plan well before I had my surgery so that I had time to get it in place beforehand. That way I knew pretty much what I was going to eat when I got home after my gastric bypass.

As well as drinking 1.5litres or 3 pints of fluids per day, my post op plan was:

Weeks 1 to 3 – fluids only

- 4 to 6 liquid meals throughout the day.
- The consistency must be lump free and able to pass through a straw
- Add extra protein to soups – you need to aim for 60 to 80g per day
- Make sure to have your Ensure nutritional drinks (dilute with equal amount of skimmed or semi-skimmed milk
- Check your weight twice weekly to make sure you are on track

Weeks 4 to 6 – purée consistency only

- 4 to 6 small meals throughout the day
- Food must be lump free and the consistency of baby food
- Add a protein rich food to every meal
- Do some light activity each day
- Make sure to have your Ensure nutritional drinks (dilute with equal amount of skimmed or semi-skimmed milk
- Check your weight twice weekly to make sure you are on track

Weeks 7 to 9 – soft consistency only

- Aim for 3 small meals a day with 1 to 2 nourishing snacks or drinks
- You can add lumpy foods but you must be able to mash them with a fork
- Add a protein rich food to every meal
- Increase the duration and intensity of your physical activity each day
- Check your weight once a week from now on

TIPS:

Use a side plate or a small bowl or ramekin

If you feel a tightness at the top of your chest STOP
EATING

Take your time – eat slowly and mindfully

DO NOT have fluids 30 minutes before or after your
food

DO NOT have fluids with your food

Try to avoid bread and red meat

Add protein powder to your meals if they are low in
protein

Post Op – Weeks 1 to 3

You can only have liquids for these first 3 weeks. Plain and simple.

During week 1 it's best to stick to clear liquids if you can. Remember you're recovering from surgery and you may well feel or even be sick.

Your tiny pouch will probably only manage a PP (Pouch Portion) of around 1 tablespoon at any one time of clear liquids.

Suggested Clear Liquids are:
Water
Sugar free squash.
Diluted sugar free juice
Still unsweetened flavoured water
Broth & broth based soups – made with Bovril,
Vegetable Stock or Chicken Bouillon or home-made
Decaffeinated tea or coffee
Sugar free ice lollies/tip-tops
Nutritional protein shakes (provided by your GP or bariatric team), diluted 50/50 with skimmed or semi-skimmed milk

All fluids should be free of all lumps and be runny enough to pass through a straw – not that you should eat through a straw. You can if you like, but I found that I was already suffering from painful trapped wind and sucking in extra air didn't help.

IMPORTANT: Don't forget to take your multivitamins and minerals every day.

During weeks 2 and 3 you have a little more choice. I remember being very nervous about eating food again even if it was mainly soup.

Take it slowly - that's very important.
Your new pouch fills up quickly but empties slowly.

You need to measure out a PP of 1 to 2 tablespoons for each meal. Sometimes it was too much for my pouch. Sometimes it was fine.

Things you can have:
Protein shakes (with 20 – 30 grams of protein in them)
High Protein Soups – tinned are fine or home-made if you feel up to it
Low fat creamy soups, strained of all lumps
Meat, fish or bean soups blended and watered down with clear broth or stock
Sugar Free Jelly
Low-fat no added sugar yoghurt (Greek has more protein)

Frozen low-fat no added sugar yoghurt – nice if you've had your surgery in the summer months
Weetabix, porridge oats or ready-brek watered down with semi-skimmed, skimmed or soy milk to a pouring consistency

TIP: Cooking, liquidising and freezing your soups into pouch portions is very handy and time saving. (I also kept a selection of pouch portions in the fridge in small microwavable containers.)

You should try to have 4 to 6 small meals or pouch portions each day, (a couple of tablespoons per meal) – imagine your new pouch as being around the size of an egg cup so this will be your pouch portion.

You'll probably only be able to manage a couple of spoonfuls to start with. Just take it slowly – your pouch will tell you when it's had enough.

IMPORTANT: Because you're only having tiny amounts, you need to make sure you add extra protein to your pouch portions at every meal. It's really important as it's a building block for muscle and tissue so it will help your wounds to heal properly, both inside and out.

Protein also gives you more energy, helps you lose fat not muscle, and gives you more post-meal satisfaction because protein digests slowly giving you the feeling of fullness for longer.

You need to make sure that you get at least 60 to 80g of protein every day after surgery – and for the rest of your life!

TIP: Plan your meals a week ahead using the meal planner template at the end of this book

WAYS TO INCREASE YOUR PROTEIN:
Get additional protein in your meals by adding mincemeat or beans to your soups, but remember to blend at this stage. No lumps allowed.

Add 4-5 tablespoons of skimmed milk powder or protein powder to a pint of skimmed or semi skimmed milk to make your own fortified milk and use this on your cereals and in your tea and coffee.

Have milky snacks like low fat/low sugar yoghurt and custard.

Your bariatric team may have given you some ready mixed nutritional drinks/meal replacements like "Fortsip" or "Fortimel" to take home which are very high in protein, vitamins and minerals. You will need to dilute them with equal amounts of skimmed or semi-skimmed milk to make them the right consistency as they're very thick.

You should aim to have ½ a bottle once or twice a day.

TIP: Your tastes may change – if something you loved before makes you nauseated, avoid it! You can always try it again at a later stage. I couldn't eat eggs without being sick even though they were one of my favourite foods prior to my op. Now, 8 months later, I can eat them again. Go figure?

THE LIQUIDS BEFORE, DURING AND AFTER MEALS RULE:

It's all about the timing!
The 30 minute rule is very important.

When you have a drink you must wait 30 minutes BEFORE you can eat your pouch portion.

You must NOT drink with your meal.

You must wait 30 minutes AFTER eating before you can drink

TIP: Always carry a bottle of still water with you everywhere you go

Stage Two – Weeks 4 To 6 – Puree

By this stage you should hopefully be feeling more like yourself and the constant chore of drinking and eating should have become easier.

Use this time to recognise that you aren't actually hungry, but just craving for foods from your old life out of habit. Drink some water, go for a walk – just do something that will keep you occupied until the craving goes away.

Again, plan your puree meals ahead using the template at the end of this book.

Your pureed food should be the consistency of baby food – however, don't be tempted to eat baby food as they don't have enough nutrients in them.

TIP: HOW TO PUREE FOODS

- Chop your chosen food into tiny pieces
- Add some liquid, (broth, gravy or skimmed/semi-skimmed milk)
- Puree in a blender or mash with a fork until smooth
- This is where a blender comes in handy

You can have (Pouch Portions of ¼ cup or 4 tablespoons):

Fat-free Refried Beans

Kidney Beans (or baked, pureed)

Chilli

Blended Soups (high protein ones)

Shredded Cheese (low-fat and melted)

Mashed low fat cottage cheese

Weetabix, porridge or ready-brek with fortified milk, (to a thicker texture than when on the liquid stage)

Low fat/low sugar yoghurt , (without fruit chunks)

Pureed white fish/meat/vegetarian food,(just have what you would normally have and blend it to a puree using a little broth/stock)

Creamed/pureed vegetables (potatoes, carrots, butternut squash etc. but avoid broccoli, cauliflower and other fibrous veggies at this stage)

Pureed stews/casseroles

Stewed apples with custard, (use artificial sweetener)

Pureed spaghetti bolognaise

Pureed Quorn

Scrambled eggs or egg substitute

Tinned tuna in brine mashed well

Mashed tinned fruit in own juice

Pureed fruit - peaches, apricots, pears or melons , (avoid pineapple as it is too acidic and has way too much sugar for your pouch)

Mashed bananas

Tomato juice

ALL stage 2 and 3 foods

IMPORTANT: Make sure you have protein at every meal. Protein creates fullness and is essential to your weight loss and healing.

TIP: Always eat the important protein portion of your food first as you will get full very quickly. So if you eat your mash first for example, you won't be able to manage your mashed white fish.

IMPORTANT: Don't forget to stay hydrated by constantly sipping throughout the day. You need to aim for a minimum of 1.5 litres or 3 pints every day, but make sure you observe the 30 minute rule!

EXERCISE: You can start doing some light activity each day; say a gentle 10 to 20 minute walk

Stage Three – Weeks 7 To 9
Soft Foods

Again, it's important to plan your soft meals ahead using the template at the end of this book.

Try to get into the habit of having 3 meals per day even if you're not hungry. It helps with your weight loss in the long run. But I never eat breakfast I hear you cry! Welcome to your new life - now you do.

You can start adding lumpy soft foods to your menu that can easily be mashed with a fork.

Your food should be of a soft consistency – not quite baby food but not solid.

Cook up some soft meals such as such as scrambled eggs, baked beans, minced meat, cottage pie, shepherd's pie, Bolognese sauce, fish in sauce/fish pie or use Soft ready meals. They are really handy when you don't want or have time to cook.

Chew each mouthful really well and stop between each one.

TIP: Only have food you can easily eat with a spoon or fork – if you need a knife it's not soft enough!

As your food is more solid you should be aiming to have 3 small meals which always include a protein rich food and 1 to 2 nourishing drinks/ snacks per day.

Snack ideas are low fat cottage cheese, low sugar/fat yoghurt, sugar free mousse, sugar free custard, fromage frais, stewed soft or tinned fruit, and low fat rice pudding.

You still need to have your 1.5 litres, (3 pints) of fluids a day to keep dehydration at bay!

You can have (Pouch Portion of ½ to 1 cup or 8 to 16 tablespoons):
All fish and shellfish
Turkey breast/chicken breast
Eggs – hard boiled, soft boiled or poached
Low fat deli meats
Low fat cheese
Cottage cheese – low fat
Baked potatoes, sweet potatoes or yams
Boiled pasta or noodles
Boiled rice
Soft fresh fruits – apples, pears, bananas etc.
Soft and/or cooked veggies
Egg Custard – no pastry
Low fat low sugar yoghurt – Greek has more protein
ALL stage 2 to 6 foods

IMPORTANT: As before, always eat your protein first and don't forget the 30 minute liquids rule!

TIPS:

If you're struggling to get in your 60 to 80g per day you can still top yourself up by having a protein shake like slim fast or shops own brand.

Stay away from red meat, bread, pasta, raw fruit and veg – you can have it soon I promise.

Don't force yourself to finish everything on your plate. I struggled with this at first as I was bought up to clear my plate before I could leave the table, starving children in Africa etc. You know how it goes.

Eat slowly but don't graze. Your meal should take no longer than 15 minutes to finish. 30 minutes plus can lead to grazing.

Constipation is a very common problem, but is easily solved by simply upping your liquid intake. Drink 2 litres of fluid instead of 1.5, and increase your fibre intake; so have porridge for breakfast or eat more fruit and veg.

For me, a gentle potter around the kitchen in the morning just after my first cup of green tea, doing my normal kitchen routine is all that's needed. Gravity, along with the warm liquid travelling through my pouch and gut stimulates my intestines into action.

Stage Four – From Week 10 & For Life

Pouch Pain and Vomiting – A Nasty Double-Act

Unfortunately this happened quite often during my early weeks of post op, when I wasn't sure when my pouch was full.

I ate too much.

It's as simple as that.

I eventually learned through trial, error and mindful eating that the tight feeling in my chest was my pouch telling me it'd had enough, and not to eat that next ½ a spoon of food because if I did I'd regret it.

Ignore your pouch at your peril!

Occasionally it happens to me now when I'm eating something I really enjoy. Mindful eating goes out the window and I revert back to my old eating habits and I wolf my food down far too quickly.

And hey presto! That nasty double-act, Pain and Vomiting are back with a vengeance.

All I can describe it as is a sharp, painful feeling at the top of my chest where my new pouch lives. Sometimes it goes away on its own, (rarely if I'm honest). Most of the time I end up being sick. Losing all of that delicious, precious protein I had been so keen to scoff just a few minutes earlier.

Ways to avoid this nasty double-act are:

EAT MINDFULLY – take your time to taste and savour your food
STOP as soon as you get a tight feeling at the top of your chest
Check the size of your **POUCH PORTIONS** – they should now be no less than ½ a cup or 8 tablespoons and no more than 1 to 1 ½ cups or 8 to 12 fluid ounces. Use small side plates and small bowls or ramekins.
DON'T take fluids and food at the same time – always leave 30 minutes before and after meals
Watch out for **POORLY TOLERATED FOODS** e.g. bread, rice, and red meats. Sometimes your pouch can stomach them, (pardon the pun) and sometimes, for no apparent reason, it can't.

DUMPING SYNDROME
I've been extremely lucky in that I've never actually experienced it. And I don't want to either! Because everyone I've spoken to says once you've experienced dumping you'll never want to experience it again.

So if you want to avoid the unpleasant dumping syndrome after bariatric surgery, its best to avoid sugary and refined foods like white flour, bread and pastries, high sugar fruit and juice.

But beware – high fat can also cause dumping.

You feel very ill within around 15 to 30 minutes of eating. You experience stomach pain and cramps at first, then symptoms of vomiting, diarrhoea, palpitations and light headedness to name but a few.

Does it mean you can never have dessert or sweets again?

No – I think you just have to learn to manage with much smaller portions.

What Medication Can I Take For Pain Relief?
The short answer is only **PARACETAMOL.**

It works surprisingly well as now everything is absorbed into your system much quicker and you're much lighter – all tablets work better now that you're not morbidly obese.

WARNING: NEVER EVER TAKE NSAIDS UNLESS ARRANGED BY YOUR BARIATRIC TEAM!
(Non-steroidal anti-inflammatory drugs)
I'm not saying this to scare you but they can eat a hole through your stomach even if you only take them once.

The main types of NSAIDs include:
ibuprofen
naproxen
diclofenac
celecoxib
mefenamic acid
etoricoxib
indometacin
aspirin – even baby aspirin
NSAIDs can be sold under these names or brand names.

It's up to you to check the packaging as other medications can contain them. Even gels and creams that you rub in for joint pain can't be used as the NSAIDS are systemic, which means they travel through your skin, into your blood stream and so into your pouch. You have to take charge of your health and life and it's important you know what medications will damage your new pouch.

As I said earlier, I'm not medically trained, but I know a couple of people from Bariatric Groups I'm on who ended up in intensive care after NSAIDS ate a hole through their pouch/sleeve!

You also need to be proactive with this information when it comes to your Dentist or Podiatrist (or any other healthcare professional for that matter).

Although bariatric surgery is becoming more and more common, they are not trained in bariatric patient care. So they may well tell you ibuprofen is fine after a dental or foot procedure to stop pain and reduce swelling.

Take charge and say you'll take Paracetamol as you've had bariatric surgery and can't take NSAIDS.

You're allowed to say NO.

It's your body and your health that are at risk at the end of the day, not theirs.

Hot Lemon Cold Remedy

I recently came down with a nasty winter's cold and as I couldn't use cold and flu remedies from over the counter anymore, (because they contain NSAIDS) I decided to make my own soothing drink.

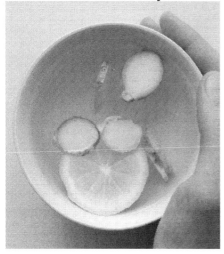

Ingredients:

Boiling water
Fresh lemon, sliced
Fresh ginger, sliced
1 Sweetener tablet if desired

METHOD
Place a couple of slices of lemon and ginger into a mug
Fill the mug with boiling water over and leave to steep.
Add sweetener to taste
Don't be tempted to eat the lemon slices prior to the soft food stage!

Alcohol and your new plumbing

Should you drink alcohol after bariatric surgery?

It's best to keep alcohol out of your diet completely if possible. Here's why:

With part of your stomach removed, (or bypassed) you can't metabolize alcohol as well.

People – bariatric patients or not – get drunk quicker on an empty stomach because the alcohol passes more quickly into the small intestines (it's not slowed down by food). With a smaller or bypassed stomach less food is there to slow down the alcohol. This is worsened by the fact that most bariatric patients observe the 30 minute drink/food rule. As a result you get intoxicated faster making you more likely to do something you'll regret like eating things you shouldn't, drunken driving, etc.

Procedures that bypass the connection between your stomach and small intestine no longer have that barrier to slow down the passing of fluids. As a result, the alcohol passes straight into your small intestines.

The sugar and carbs in alcohol are empty calories too so you risk weight gain.

As a weight loss surgery patient, you have a greater risk of alcohol-related health problems such as acid reflux, gastric and oesophageal cancer, liver damage and heart problems. And to top it all off, bariatric patients are also more susceptible to alcoholism due to addiction transfer – swapping their food addiction for alcohol.

So should you drink alcohol after bariatric surgery? If you decide the answer is yes here are a few tips to remember:

Like eating after weight loss surgery, alcohol intake should be done mindfully. Think to yourself, do I really want this drink, or am I just in a habit of pouring a glass of wine each night. You may find you can cut you alcohol intake without even missing it.

Try non-alcoholic wines etc. which let you to feel part of the social scene without the unwelcome side effects.

Choose wisely if you decide to drink. Opt for lower calorie drinks like as vodka with soda water and lime. Drink lots of non-alcoholic fluid in between to prevent dehydration.

Don't let alcohol replace meals. While trying to keep food and fluids separate, it's easy to skip a meal, but it's important that this doesn't happen.

THINGS THAT AREN'T ESSENTIAL TO HAVE BUT ARE LIFESAVERS IF YOU DO

You may well already have some of these items of equipment in your kitchen already which is great.
If you don't then I suggest you get them if you can as they will save you endless time and effort during the entire post op eating stages, especially the early ones of fluids and purees.

By the way I'm not endorsing these brands – they're just the ones that I use and work for me.

Bullet Type Blender
I got myself a Breville Blend-Active VBL096 Blender for around £40 prior to my bypass. It came with four bottles - great to store my soups etc. in the fridge. And it could crush ice which came in handy for fruit smoothies in the summer. I've actually just given it away to my sister who is just about to have her bariatric surgery, and also, I tend to use my stick blender more now that I'm at the "Eating for Life stage".

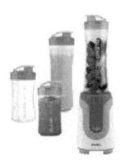

Breville Blend-Active VBL096 Blender

There are cheaper ones on the market for around £10 each and obviously much more expensive ones, but as long as they blend to a smooth consistency you'll be fine.

Stick or Hand Blender
Invest in a good stick blender as it will make light work of soups and purees. Their advantage is that there's no decanting and they can be used straight in the slow cooker or saucepan. I use a Braun Hand Held Emersion blender that I've had for years and it's still going strong.

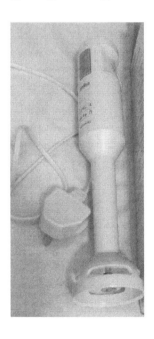

There are plenty similar ones out there and they start from around £12

Ramekin Dishes

I found that these were the easiest way to measure out a single pouch portion. I got mine from the Asda for £1 each but they're available in most stores that sell homewares.

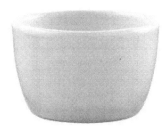

I have 8 of them and I use them to store my Pouch Portions in the fridge, freeze them, microwave and grill with them.

Ziploc Soup Bags

These are perfect for freezing broths, soups and any other meal you cook in bulk. Get them in small and large sizes, always make sure food is cool before freezing and always write on the bag what it is and the date.

Measuring Spoons & Cups

These are another great little tool that helps with getting your Pouch Portion size right. And also for some recipes you find online that are in American "Cups".

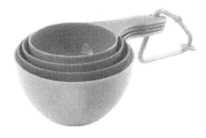

Mine are coloured plastic from the Asda, and again I've had them for years. I've got 2 sorts: Cups and Spoons, and you can pick them up from most supermarket stores for around £2 per set.

Plates & Bowls

There are of course lots of great gadgets out there for post op bariatric patients like portion control plates and bowls, but all you really need is a small side plate and bowl - much cheaper.

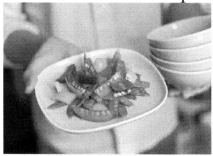

TIPS: JUST IN CASE YOU'VE FORGOTTEN

Keep hydrated! To drink your 1.5litres (3 pints) per day you're going to have to sip, sip, sip all day long.

If your pee is almost clear then you're fine, but if it's dark, (and quite possibly smelly) you're dehydrated and you need to drink more!

Keep a bottle of water with you at all times.

No straws or chewing gum. They put air into your pouch, which is very uncomfortable. And you don't want to accidentally swallow the gum as it can get stuck in the opening to your pouch and may need to be surgically removed.

Don't eat and drink at the same time. Don't drink for 30 minutes before a meal and wait 30 minutes after eating.

Use smaller utensils and plates to control portions.

Use restraint when trying new foods by introducing one at a time.

Vary the food you eat to meet nutritional needs and keep it interesting.

Focus on nutrient/protein rich foods.

Take small bites about the size of your little finger nail and chew, chew, chew each mouthful mindfully

Eat slowly. Take 15 to 30 minutes to finish a meal but no longer.

Eat your protein first. It makes you feel full longer.

Avoid high-fat and fried foods.

Avoid simple sugars like sweets, cookies, cake, etc.

Don't eat too much in one sitting or you will be sick, have stabbing pains and/or stretch your new pouch.

Listen to your body and don't overeat.

Learn to tell the difference between being full and being satisfied.

From week 7 onwards make sure you have breakfast, lunch and dinner with 1 or 2 snacks.

Avoid mindless eating.

Watch less TV and take up a hobby.

Sleep more

Join a Bariatric Support Group and attend them regularly – your Bariatric Team probably have one!

Have a shopping list when you shop and only buy what's on the list.

Don't shop while you're hungry.

Be very mindful when drinking alcohol.

Use a meal planner or a food diary. Keeping track of what you eat makes you more aware of what you're putting into your pouch.

Take your multivitamins/mineral supplements and any other supplements as specified by your bariatric team.

POUCH PORTION

Recipe Section

    I. CLEAR FLUIDS

   II. FULL FLUIDS

  III. PUREES

  IV. SOFT FOODS

POUCH PORTIONS FOR LIFE

Dear PP Reader,

Here are some of my favourite recipes.
They give you protein, taste and are
really easy to make.

Enjoy!

RECIPES: WEEKS 1

CLEAR FLUIDS

If you really don't feel up to cooking your own clear broth, you can use the following instant stocks for a quick and easy liquid meal. However, liquid bouillon, pastes or stock cubes all contain quite a bit of salt unless you specifically buy the low salt versions. I did use them occasionally, I must admit.

Making your own broth will give you control over how much salt you are using and generally will taste better and contain much better nutrients.

BRANDS OF INSTANT STOCK – other brands are available…

Knorr Touch of Taste Chicken or Beef Concentrated Liquid Stock
Bisto Chicken Bouillon Paste
Knorr Chicken, Beef or Vegetable Stock Cubes
Maggi Chicken Bouillon Stock Cubes
Oxo Chicken, Beef or Vegetable Stock Cubes
Kallo Chicken, Beef or Vegetable Stock Cubes
Bovril Chicken or Beef Extract

Just add 1 teaspoon to a ramekin of boiling water and voila!

It's done and ready to drink!
If you'd like to try your hand at making your own nutritious broths though, read on...

SLOW COOKER BROTH RECIPES

(You can make these up before your surgery and freeze them in readiness for when you need them)

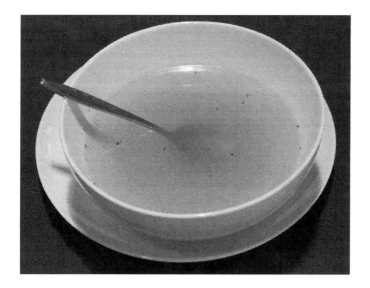

CHICKEN BROTH

Ingredients:
1.36g chicken thighs/wings, bone in and skin on
1 medium onion, coarsely chopped
5cm fresh ginger, sliced
1 teaspoon sea salt
2 bay leaves
3 litres water

METHOD

- Rinse chicken pieces then place in the bottom of slow cooker
- Add onion, ginger, sea salt, bay leaves then pour in water
- Cover and cook on low for 8-9 hours or on high for 4-5 hours
-
- Let the broth settle for 5 minutes then remove as much fat as possible from the surface using a large spoon.
-
- Discard the solids and strain the broth through
- a fine-mesh strainer or muslin cloth into a large container.
-
- Enjoy hot and refrigerate or freeze the leftovers for later.

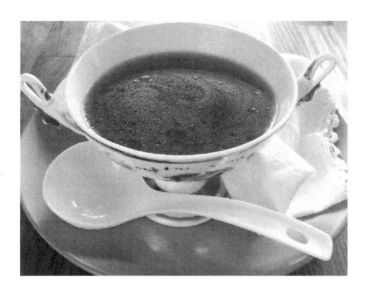

BEEF BONE BROTH

INGREDIENTS
2 carrots, roughly chopped
2 celery stalks, chopped
1 medium onion, roughly chopped
7 garlic cloves, smashed
1.36g to 1.58g of beef bones
2 bay leaves
2 tablespoons of apple cider vinegar
sea salt
3 litres water

METHOD
- Put carrots, celery, onion and garlic into a slow cooker.
- Place beef bones on top of the vegetables.
- Add bay leaves and drizzle with apple cider vinegar.

- Sprinkle a pinch of salt then add the water.
- Cover and cook on low for 8-10 hours.
- Discard the solids and strain the broth through a fine-mesh strainer or muslin cloth into a large container.
- Enjoy hot and refrigerate or freeze the leftovers for later.

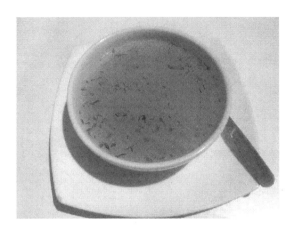

VEGETABLE BROTH

Alter it according to the ingredients you have available
Ingredients:
2 medium onions, chopped
2 to 3 carrots, chopped
3 to 4 celery stalks, chopped
1 large tomato, chopped
227g mushrooms (or mushroom stems)
4 sprigs fresh thyme (optional)
1 bay leaf
1 small bunch parsley
Salt, to taste
1 teaspoon whole peppercorns
2 to 3 litres water

METHOD
- Combine all ingredients in a 6-quart slow cooker. Cover and cook on low for 8-9 hours or on high for 4-5 hours.
- Discard the solids and strain the broth through a fine-mesh strainer into a large container.

- Enjoy hot and refrigerate or freeze the leftovers for later.

HOW TO STORE YOUR HOME-MADE BROTH

Broth freezes well so you can make it in big batches so it's readily available for enjoying on its own or in other recipes.

You can store your frozen broth for up to six months - don't forget to write the date on the Ziploc bag with a sharpie pen!

There are lots of ways to freeze broth, but here are some of my favourites.

ZIPLOC BAGS

Ladle your broth into a coffee mug or jug lined with a small Ziploc bag. Seal the bag and repeat. Put the filled bags flat in a large shallow roasting tray and pop into your freezer. Once the broth is frozen solid, remove from the tray and store back in your freezer.

SILICONE MUFFIN TRAYS

Ladle cooled broth into silicone muffin trays and freeze. Once the broth is frozen, twist the muffin tray to get the frozen broth out. Pop the frozen blocks in a large Ziploc bag and store in the freezer.

RECIPES: WEEKS 2 TO 3
FULL FLUIDS

FORTIFIED MILK

Ingredients:
4-5 tablespoons of skimmed milk powder or protein powder
570mls of skimmed or semi skimmed milk

METHOD
Mix ingredients together in a blender or with a whisk
Use on your cereals and in your tea and coffee to add extra protein

TINNED SOUPS

There's nothing wrong with using ready made soups. They;re great if you just don't have the energy or the wherewithal to cook. Just make sure you check the label for ones with high protein content. These are normally the meat, beans and lentil varieties.
I got a stock of them in prior to my surgery so that I'd have something to fall back on if need be, and they were a godsend.
Just mix 1 tin of soup to 2 tins of broth, blend until there are no lumps in sight, heat up and season to taste.

Making your own soup is really easy too though, especially if you have a hand stick blender because you just do it all in the saucepan. Here are a few of my favourites.

CLEAR SPINACH SOUP

Ingredients:
Spinach, sliced, 680g
Onions, finely chopped, 170g
Garlic, chopped, 2 tsp.
Vegetable oil, 1 tsp.
Salt and pepper, to taste

METHOD
- Heat oil in a medium-sized non-stick pan.
- Add the onions and garlic.
- Cook until the onions turn reddish-brown.
- Add the spinach.
- Cook on high heat until the spinach is bright green in colour.
- Turn the heat off.
- Add 3 cups of cold water.
- Purée this mixture in a blender.
- Pour back into the pan and bring to the boil.
- Add salt and pepper to taste and serve hot.

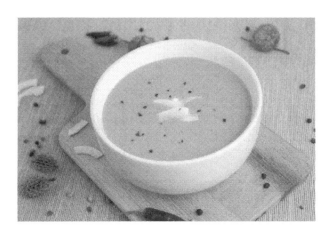

SPICED PUMPKIN SOUP

Ingredients:
Low-fat cooking spray oil
1 large onion, chopped
3 cloves garlic, crushed
5 cm piece fresh ginger, grated
2 tsp medium curry powder
750g pumpkin or squash flesh, peeled and cubed
400g tin reduced fat coconut milk
400 ml vegetable stock/bouillon
Salt and freshly ground black pepper

METHOD
- Spray a large saucepan with low-fat cooking spray oil and heat
- Add chopped onions and cook for 3 – 4 minutes until softened
- Add ginger, garlic and curry powder and cook for 1 minute
- Add the cubed pumpkin or squash, coconut milk and stock

- Bring to boil then reduce heat and simmer for 10-12 minutes until pumpkin is tender
- Puree with a hand "stick" blender or food processor until smooth
- Season to taste
- Reheat and serve hot

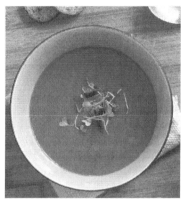

BEEF & TOMATO SOUP

Ingredients:
1 400g tin cream of Tomato Soup
1 400g tin Beef Consommé
500mls water
1 teaspoon Worcestershire sauce
1 Tablespoon lemon juice
Salt and ground black pepper

METHOD
- Empty all ingredients into a saucepan
- Heat until boiling
- Turn down the heat and simmer for 5 minutes
- Serve

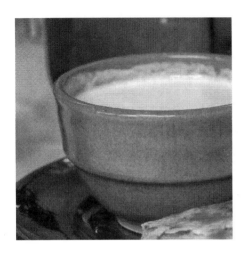

WHITE BEAN SOUP
Serves 4

Ingredients:
1 400g tin white kidney or cannellini beans rinsed and drained
250ml chicken broth
2 tablespoons chopped onion
1 tablespoons olive oil
1 garlic clove, minced
60ml evaporated milk
1 teaspoon minced fresh parsley
½ teaspoon salt
½ teaspoon dried thyme
¼ teaspoon cayenne pepper

METHOD
- In a saucepan cook onions in olive oil over a medium heat until tender
- Add the garlic and sauté for 1 minute

- Stir in beans, chicken broth, evaporated milk, parsley, salt, thyme, and cayenne pepper
- Bring to a boil
- Reduce heat and simmer, uncovered for 12-15 minutes or until heated through. Cool slightly and blend with a stick blender or in a food processor until smooth then serve

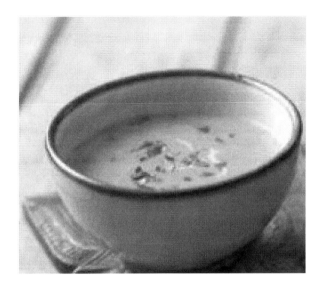

SLOW COOKER CHICKEN AND LENTIL SOUP

Ingredients:
2 Carrots
1 Bell Pepper
1 Onion
240g of barley, lentils and split peas
2 large sliced potatoes
2 cubes of vegetable stock
Chicken Breasts
2 Litres of water

METHOD

- Chop up the vegetables, slice the potato and put into the slow cooker
- Add the pulses and vegetable stock
- Cover and cook on low for 3-4 hours
- Puree with a hand "stick" blender or food processor until smooth
- Season to taste
- Reheat and serve hot

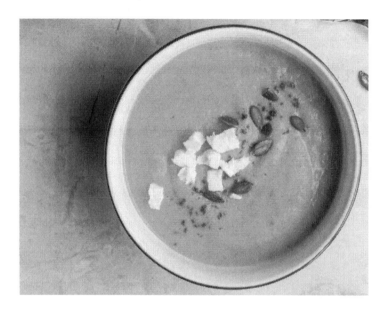

ROASTED BUTTERNUT SQUASH SOUP
Serves 8

Ingredients:
1.5kg peeled and deseeded butternut squash, cut into 3cm cubes
1 large onion, roughly chopped
2 medium carrots, peeled and chopped

1 red pepper, deseeded and cut into cubes
4 tbsp olive oil
1 tbsp clear honey
5cm piece fresh root ginger, peeled and chopped
1.5 litres pints vegetable stock
salt and ground black pepper

METHOD
- Preheat the oven to 400F/200C/180C Fan/Gas 6.
- Tip the prepared squash into a large, re-sealable freezer bag with the onion, carrots and red pepper.
- Add half the oil and salt and pepper and toss everything together until the vegetables are evenly coated.
- Tip into a large roasting tin and spread out to form a single layer.
- Roast in the oven for 40–45 minutes, or until tender and tinged brown.
- Drizzle over the honey 5 minutes before the end of cooking.
- Place a large saucepan over a medium heat
- Add the remaining oil and, when it is hot, add the ginger and fry for a minute.
- Pour in the stock and bring to the boil then stir in the roasted vegetables and add salt and pepper.
- Remove the saucepan from the heat and, using a hand blender, blend the mixture until smooth.
- Return to heat to warm through and serve hot
- Add Pumpkin seeds and cubes of goats cheese to upscale this soup to "eating for life" stage

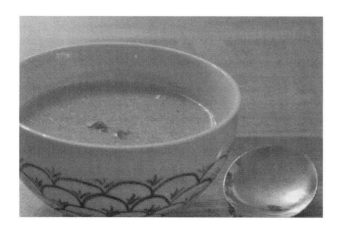

HIGH PROTEIN BROCCOLI & CHEESE SOUP

Ingredients:
680 to 907g of broccoli chopped
500ml of milk
470g of cottage cheese
1.4ltr of chicken broth
120g of flour
120g of spring onions
1 tablespoon of oregano
1 tablespoon of mustard
salt and pepper to taste

METHOD
- Put the milk, cheese and chicken broth into a large saucepan
- Cook on a low heat until the cottage cheese completely melts
- Add the remaining ingredients then simmer on a medium heat for 10 minutes
- Purée with a stick blender until it has a creamy consistency & serve hot.

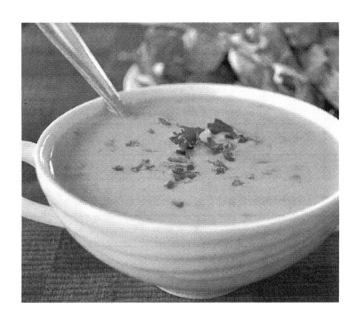

CHICKEN & MUSHROOM SOUP

Ingredients:
1 onion sliced thinly
3 gloves garlic crushed
4 cups fresh mushrooms
1 sweet potato peeled and diced
1 small yellow squash, peeled and diced
460g boneless skinless chicken breast
700ml Chicken Stock
salt & pepper
Dried Oregano & thyme or Chicken Seasoning
500ml water or broth for pureeing

METHOD
- Put all of the ingredients into a big saucepan and boil for 5 to 10 minutes until the chicken is thoroughly cooked

- Add 500ml more of broth and purée with a stick blender
- Turn down the heat to medium and simmer for 5 minutes
- Add salt and pepper to taste
- Serve hot

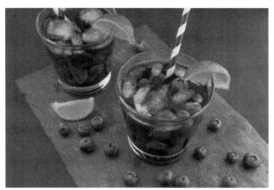

BLUEBERRY LIMEADE

Ingredients
2 cups fresh blueberries
1/3 cup freshly squeezed lime juice
6 cups water and Sweetener to taste

METHOD
- Blend blueberries, sweetener, lime juice, and 1 cup water in a blender
- Pour into a jug.
- Add remaining water and stir.
- Serve cold in a glass over ice cubes.

(NOTE: do not eat blueberries whole no matter how much you fancy one!)

RECIPES: WEEKS 4 TO 6 PUREES

I must admit I did struggle slightly with this stage and I tended to have quick and "easy" food over hand cooked "recipe" based food.

My Go-To list of "easy" foods:

Weetabix, porridge, Ready Brek with plenty of skimmed or semi-skimmed milk to make a runny consistency
Mashed banana with yogurt or custard
Very very soft cooked scrambled egg
Finely minced or pureed chicken or turkey in thin gravy
Pureed fish in a thin parsley or cheese sauce
Pureed tinned fish e.g. tuna, pilchards, salmon or mackerel in a thin tomato sauce – not oil
Soft and smooth pate or spread
Plain cottage cheese, on its own or topped with pureed fruit
Pureed mashed potato with thin gravy
Pureed tinned or very tender boiled vegetables
Fromage Frais
Smooth mousse made with milk
Mashed potato with grated cheese or cream cheese
Milky pudding like tapioca, sago or rice pudding

Pureed cauliflower cheese in cheese sauce
Pureed vegetable, bean or chicken soups
Pureed casseroles and stews to a "thinnish" consistency
Pureed Soft beans, lentils or peas
Fruit smoothies
Pureed avocado
Small portions of home-cooked or shop bought ready-meals and pureed main dishes like cottage pie, shepherd's pie, fish pie, fish-in-sauce, mild chilli con carne or their vegetarian alternatives made with quorn
Sorbets
Silken or smooth tofu

Don't feel bad about using the "easy" foods, but do try to make sure they contain protein.

You can do this by adding a scoop of protein powder to most of these "easy" foods. And of course, always make low-fat and low-sugar choices.

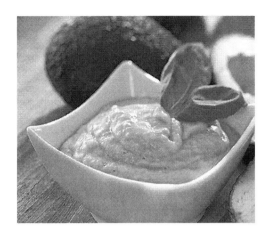

CHICKEN AVOCADO & POTATO PUREE

Ingredients:
1 small potato peeled and cut into chunks
50 g/2oz skinless boneless chicken thigh or breast
1/2 ripe avocado peeled and stoned
2 tsp skimmed milk
salt and pepper to taste

METHOD
- Steam the potato and chicken together for 25-30 minutes
- Place in a blender with the avocado, milk and salt and pepper and puree to the desired consistency (thin with more milk if you want a runnier puree)

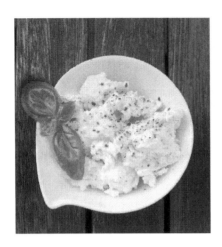

CRAB SPREAD

Ingredients:
60g fat-free cream cheese
120g fat-free cottage cheese
60g light mayonnaise
1 Tbsp. Bari-Clear Protein Powder
60g cup shredded 2% cheddar cheese
1 Tbsp. hot mustard
1/4 tsp. Horseradish
1 tsp. garlic powder
1 tin shredded crab meat

METHOD
- Place cream cheese, cottage cheese, and crab meat into a food processor/blender and blend until smooth.
- Mix in the rest of the ingredients by hand.
- Heat in microwave 3-5 minutes.
- Let cool for 5 minutes before eating.

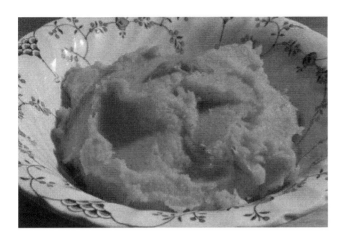

PUREED VEGETABLES

Ingredients:
Any peeled root veggies you have but a few of my favourites are
Peas & Fresh Mint
Butternut Squash
Parsnip
Carrot
(Avoid putting potatoes and some starchy squash in a blender as it just creates a sticky mess – they will need to be hand mashed)

METHOD
- Cook the vegetable of your choice fully - not al dente, or just barely fork-tender. Heat them until they're fully soft all around, but not yet waterlogged
- Once fully cooked (boiled, baked or steamed) puree in a blender or food processor.
- Season with salt and pepper
- Mix in cream, crème fresh or butter and serve

LEMON RICOTTA CRÈME

Ingredients:
1 425g packet of low fat ricotta cheese
Zest of a lemon
1-2 teaspoons of lemon extract
1 ½ teaspoons vanilla extract
4 pkts of splenda or stevia

METHOD
Put all ingredients into a blender and puree until smooth
Spoon into a ramekin, mini kilner jar or similar and store in the fridge until ready to serve

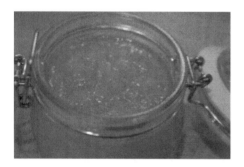

PUREED FRUIT

Peaches, raspberries, strawberries, blueberries, apricots, apples, pears or melons are just some of the fruits that can be pureed and used as a tasty topping to cottage cheese or yoghurt. You can even eat it on its own within moderation.
Try to avoid pineapple if you can as it is too acidic and has way too much sugar for your pouch.

Here is the recipe for Applesauce but you can use any fruit you like:

- Peel, core and cut 2 apples into slices/chunks
- Place slices or chunks into a pan with just enough water to slightly cover apples and boil/steam until tender; reserve the cooking water for thinning your puree later on
- Apples can be mashed with a potato masher once cooked to achieve a smooth applesauce or you can put them into a blender to puree
- Add the reserved water as necessary to achieve a smooth puree
- If you want something sweet, add sugar free syrup, (any flavour) at this stage too
- Freeze Pouch Portions in *ice cube trays* and once frozen, remove from tray and pop into Ziploc bags to store until needed in the freezer

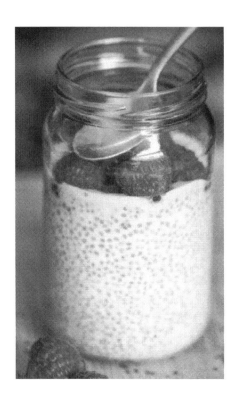

VANILLA & ALMOND CHIA BREAKFAST PUDDING

(This is still one of my favourite breakfast recipes)

Ingredients

500mls unsweetened almond milk, home-made or shop bought (see recipe below)
8 tablespoons chia seeds
1/2 teaspoon vanilla extract
1-2 tablespoons sugar free maple syrup or raw honey
Fruit for topping (whatever you fancy)
Chopped Almonds or again whatever you like for the topping

METHOD

- Mix the almond milk, chia seeds, vanilla and sweetener in a bowl.
- Stir well until combined and the mixture starts to thicken.
- Store covered in the fridge overnight (or for at least an hour).
- Stir well before serving (add a drop of water if the pudding is too thick).
- Top with fresh fruit and nuts of your choice - This keeps up to 5 days in the fridge.

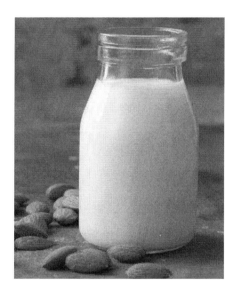

HOME-MADE UNSWEETENED ALMOND MILK

Ingredients
16 tablespoons almond flour or ground almonds
1 litre water

METHOD

- Put almonds in a bowl and cover them with water. Leave to soak for at least three hours, but preferably overnight.
- Drain the almond and put in a blender with 4 cups of water and blend for one minute.
- Strain the almond milk through a fine mesh strainer or muslin cloth into a container, cover and refrigerate for up to five days.

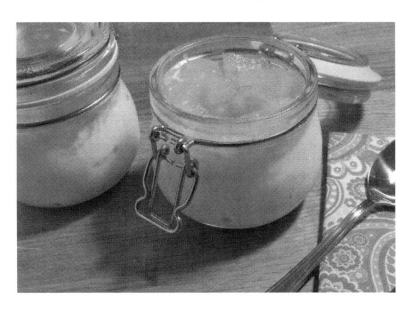

COTTAGE CHEESE WITH POACHED PEARS

Ingredients:
355g plain low fat cottage cheese
1 ½ teaspoons vanilla extract
4 pkts of splenda or stevia
2 scoops unflavoured protein powder
6 tablespoons pureed pears (or fruit of your choice) for topping

METHOD

- Put all ingredients except pureed fruit into bowl and mix well until semi- smooth
- Spoon into 6 ramekins, mini kilner jars or similar and top with pureed fruit then chill in the fridge until ready to serve

RECIPES: WEEKS 7 TO 9
SOFT FOODS

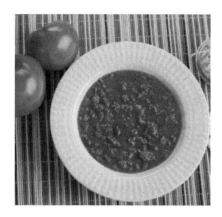

NANCY'S CHILLI BEEF

Ingredients:
1 tbsp oil
1 large onion finely diced
1 red pepper, chopped
2 garlic cloves, peeled and crushed
1 heaped tsp hot chilli powder (or 1 level tbsp of mild)
1 tsp paprika
1 tsp ground cumin
500g lean minced beef
1 beef stock cube
300ml hot water
400g tin chopped tomatoes
½ tsp dried marjoram
1 tsp granulated sweetener
2 tbsp tomato purée

410g can red kidney beans
soured cream, to serve
2 tablespoons unsweetened cocoa powder
Salt and pepper, to taste

METHOD

- Heat oil in a pan on the hob over a medium heat until hot
- Add the onions and cook for about 5 minutes until soft
- Add garlic, red pepper, chilli powder, paprika and ground cumin and cook for 5 minutes, stirring occasionally
- Add the minced beef and fry for 5 minutes until the mince is browned
- Crumble the beef stock cube into 300ml hot water and add to the mince along with the chopped tomatoes, dried marjoram, sweetener, tomato purée and salt and pepper
- Bring to the boil then turn down the heat and simmer for 20 minutes, stirring occasionally
- Now add the kidney beans and cocoa powder, stir well and bring to the boil again for another 10 minute
- Turn off the heat and leave your chilli to stand for 10 minutes with the lid on
- Serve piping hot

Toppings:

- Greek Yogurt
- Sour cream
- Shredded cheese
- Jalapenos

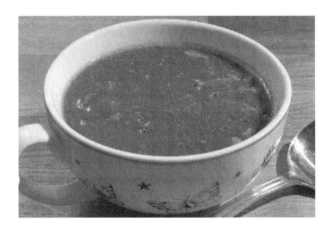

EASY BEEF CASSEROLE

Ingredients:
1 to 1.5 lbs stewing beef cut into chunks
1 onion, diced
1 large Potato, diced
2 carrots, chopped
2 celery sticks, chopped
8 oz mushrooms, chopped
3 garlic cloves, minced
3 tablespoons tomato paste
1 tablespoon Worcester sauce
1 tsp rosemary
1tsp thyme

1 Bay leaf
Salt and pepper to taste
900mls beef bone broth, (or stock made from cubes or bouillon)
NOTE: you can use any vegetables you like

METHOD

- This is so simple – just throw everything into your slow cooker and cook for 6 to 8 hours on low.
- If you like a thicker textured casserole, add 2 heaped tablespoons of pearl barley or lentils for the last 30 minutes of cooking which will also add to the casserole's fibre and protein content.

NOTE: You can prep it the night before, put it in the fridge, and then pop it on next morning.

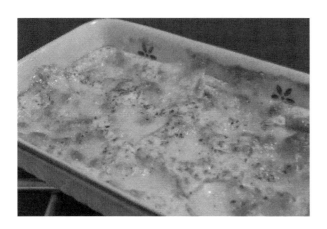

NO PASTA CHEESE LASAGNE

Ingredients
180g fat free or low fat cottage or ricotta cheese
60ml marinara or spaghetti sauce
1/4 tsp oregano
1/4 tsp basil
2 egg whites
60g low fat mozzarella cheese

METHOD

- Mix cottage or ricotta cheese, egg whites, oregano, basil together and place in an oven proof dish.
- Pour marinara sauce on top of mixture and top with mozzarella cheese.
- Bake it in the oven @ 450F/230C/210Fan/Gas 8 for about 20 minutes or heat in the microwave until hot and bubbly.

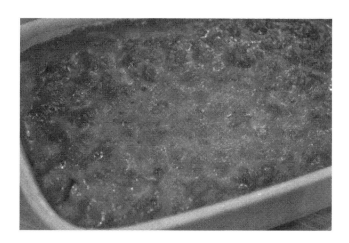

SPICY MEXICAN CASSEROLE

Ingredients
1 lb minced turkey
1 small courgette diced
1 small yellow onion diced
1 garlic clove minced
1 pkg taco seasoning
10 oz black beans drained and rinsed
8 oz fat-free refried beans canned
8 oz tomatoes & chillies canned
2 c Mexican blend cheese

METHOD

- Preheat oven to 350F/180C/Gas4/160CFan
- Spray a pan with non-stick cooking spray and put in the oven to heat up
- Sauté the vegetables and garlic until softened
- Drain any excess liquid and transfer to a bowl with beans, tomatoes and chillies

- Brown minced turkey, drain and add to bowl with taco seasoning and mix well
- Transfer mixture to a large casserole dish
- Spread fat free refried beans on top (heat for 1 minute in a microwave first)
- Top with cheese and bake in oven for 30 minutes or until the cheese has melted and is slightly browned
- Cool 10-15 minutes before slicing and serving

Tuna Salad

Ingredients:
1 tin of flaked tuna in brine
2 tablespoons of plain Greek yoghurt
½ cucumber skinned and finely diced
Sprinkle of dill
Salt and pepper to taste

METHOD
- Drain the water off the tuna and place tuna in a bowl
- Add all other ingredients and mix well – add more or less yoghurt to your taste, depending on desired consistency
- Chill for 20 minutes then serve

   NOTE: When on soft food you can used thin slices of cucumber as crackers for your tuna topping.

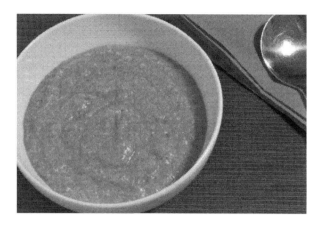

SLOW COOKER CHICKEN CURRY

Ingredients:
1 onion peeled & quartered
5 garlic cloves peeled
5cm ginger root sliced roughly
2 tomatoes, quartered
I tsp salt
1/2 tsp cayenne pepper
2 tsp turmeric
1 tsp garam masala, can buy ready mixed or use this recipe
120g greek yogurt
680g of chicken, skinned
1 bag of baby spinach
1 5cm piece cinnamon stick
4 green cardamom
2 whole cloves

METHOD
- In a food processor blend together, everything except the chicken, spinach and whole spices, to make a smooth paste.
- Put the chicken pieces into a slow cooker and pour over the paste
- Add the whole spices
- Chop up the spinach and add during the last hour of cooking
- Cook on low for 8 hours or high for 4 until chicken is tender
- Serve hot

Southern Bean Dip

Ingredients:
1 400g tin baked beans, drained
80g mild salsa
60g coriander
120g grated Hot Mexican cheese

METHOD

- Preheat the oven to 400F/200C/180c Fan/Gas 6
- Using a stick blender or food processor pulse the beans and salsa until semi smooth
- Add coriander and pulse until some texture remains
- Pour into a baking dish and top with cheese
- Cook in oven for 25 to 30 minutes
- Serve hot

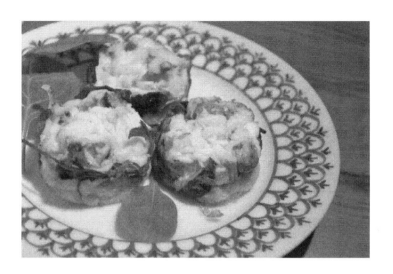

HIGH PROTEIN SPINACH & CHEESE BREAKFAST BITES

Ingredients:
1 cup fresh spinach leaves
2 tomatoes, diced
4 rashers bacon, grilled (or cooked ham or salmon)
4oz cheese, grated
8 egg whites
Salt & pepper to taste

METHOD

- Preheat oven 350F/180C/160c Fan/Gas 4
- Spray muffin trays with oil
- Line bottom of each well with fresh spinach
- Add teaspoon of tomatoes and teaspoon of bacon to each well

- Pour whisked egg whites into each well then top with cheese
- Sprinkle with salt and pepper
- Cook in oven for 15 minutes
- Serve hot or cold
- (makes 6 large or 12 small)

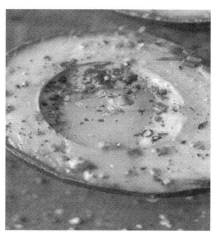

AVOCADO BREAKFAST EGGS

Ingredients:
1 ripe avocado cut in half and de-stoned
Lemon juice
2 eggs
Fresh chives, chopped finely
Salt & pepper to taste

METHOD
- Preheat oven 425F/220c/gas7/200fan
- Lightly spray oil onto a baking sheet
- Scoop out around 2tbsp of avocado flesh, or enough to create small wells in the middle of each avocado half.
- Gently crack an egg into each well keeping the yolk intact
- Season with salt and pepper to taste.
- Place on baking tray and cook for around 15-18 minutes or until the egg whites have set but the yolks are still fairly runny
- Top with a few chives and serve while hot

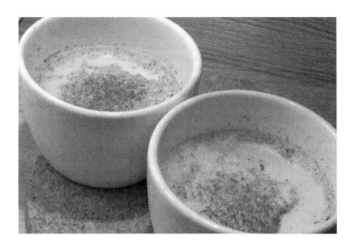

EGG CUSTARD

Ingredients:
236ml milk
One 340g tin evaporated milk
4 large eggs
19g Splenda or Stevia
2 teaspoons vanilla extract
Freshly grated nutmeg

METHOD
- Preheat oven 400F/200C/180c Fan/Gas 6
- Put 6 ramekins in a large roasting tray
- Place the milk, evaporated milk, eggs, Splenda and vanilla in a bowl and blend with a stick blender, (or use a food processor) until smooth
- Pour mixture into ramekins
- Grate nutmeg on top of each one
- Pour boiling water from a kettle into the pan until it comes to half way up the ramekin dishes

- Place in the oven and bake for 25 to 30 minutes until just set in the centre
- Do not remove from the oven until they are set
- Carefully remove from the oven and water bath
- Place each egg custard onto a paper towel or t-towel to cool then put in the fridge
- Serve chilled

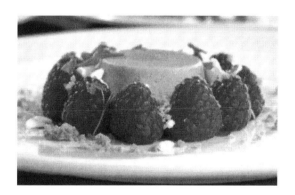

RASPBERRY JELLY MOUSSE

Ingredients:
1 small box/packet sugar free Raspberry Jelly (or whatever flavour you like)
118ml of water
2 pots of low fat/low sugar Raspberry Greek yogurt (or whatever flavour you like but it's best to match the yoghurt to the jelly)
2 scoops unflavoured protein powder
Fresh Raspberries to decorate
METHOD
- Heat water until it's warm but not boiling.
- In a mixing bowl, empty sugar-free jelly mix, pour the water over it and stir

- Add the yoghurt and protein powder to the bowl and whisk until smooth
- Pour into 4 ramekins and leave to set

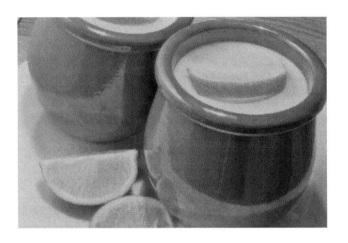

LIME MOUSSE

Ingredients:
1 small box/packet sugar-free key lime jelly
60ml cup of water
355g plain Greek yogurt
2 scoops unflavoured protein powder

METHOD
- Heat the water until it's hot but not boiling
- Put the jelly powder into a bowl and pour the hot water on top of the crystals
- Put the plain yogurt and protein powder into the bowl and blend
- Pour mixture into 6 ramekins and leave to set

RECIPES: WEEKS 10

POUCH PORTIONS FOR LIFE

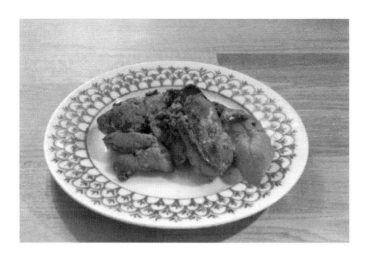

CHICKEN LIVERS IN GARLIC BUTTER

Ingredients:
1 Tub of frozen chicken livers, fully defrosted
1 tablespoon butter
Dash of olive oil
1 teaspoon crushed garlic
Salt & pepper to taste

METHOD
- Wash and dry the chicken livers
- Heat a small frying pan on the hob over a medium heat
- Add the oil and butter and melt

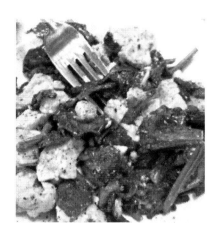

CHICKEN GARLIC PARMESAN

Ingredients:
3 tbsp. butter
6 cloves minced garlic
2 chicken breasts-chopped into bite size pieces
salt to taste
¼-1/2 cup grated parmesan cheese
2 cups fresh spinach

METHOD
- Gently Sauté garlic in butter for a minute or two
- Add chicken pieces, salt, and fry until thoroughly cooked - make sure that the chicken is coated with butter and garlic
- Add the parmesan cheese and stir until the chicken is coated
- Add the spinach and cook until it's wilted and serve hot

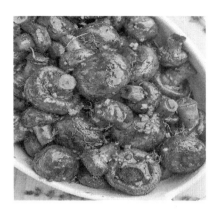

ROASTED GARLIC MUSHROOMS IN BALSAMIC SOY SAUCE

Ingredients:
2 pounds mushrooms
1 tablespoon oil
3 tablespoons balsamic vinegar
2 tablespoons soy sauce (or tamari)
3 cloves garlic, chopped
1/2 teaspoon thyme, chopped
Salt and pepper to taste

METHOD
- Preheat your oven to 400F/200C/gas6/180Fan
- Toss the mushrooms in the oil, balsamic vinegar, soy sauce, garlic, thyme, salt and pepper
- Arrange mushrooms in a single layer on a baking sheet
- Roast in the oven until the mushrooms are tender, approx. 20 minutes, stirring about half way through.
- Serve piping hot

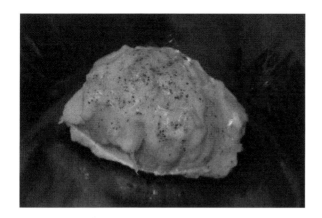

CHICKEN BREAST WITH BACON AND CHEESE

Ingredients:
1 small chicken breast
1 rasher of streaky bacon
1 tbsp grated mature cheddar cheese
Salt & pepper to taste

METHOD
- Preheat oven 350F/180C/160cFan/Gas4
- Wash and dry the chicken breast
- Wrap bacon around it
- Top with cheese
- Wrap in tin foil – create a little parcel sealed at both ends
- Place on a baking tray and cook in the oven for 40 minutes
- Tip in the chicken livers and garlic then cook for 3 or 4 minutes until brown on both sides, (be careful as they may spit!)
- Serve immediately.

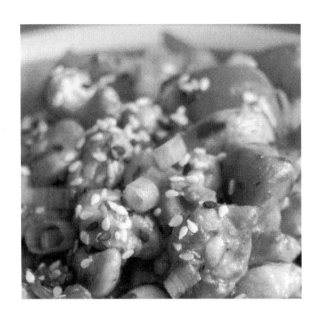

CASHEW CHICKEN

Ingredients:
3 raw chicken thighs boneless, skinless chopped into
bite size pieces
2 tbsp oil for cooking
1/4 cup cashews
1/2 medium Green Bell Pepper diced
1/2 tsp ground ginger
1 tbsp rice wine vinegar
1 1/2 tbsp soy sauce
½ tbsp. chilli oil
1 tbsp minced garlic
1 tbsp Sesame Oil
1 tbsp Sesame Seeds
1 tbsp spring onions chopped quite finely
1/4 medium white onion diced
 Salt + Pepper

METHOD

- Heat a frying pan on a low heat and toast the cashews for 8 minutes or until they start to go brown then place them on one side
- Turn up the heat, add the oil and once up to temperature fry the chicken until cooked through.
- Add the pepper, onions, garlic, chilli oil, ginger, salt and pepper. Cook for 2 to 3 minutes
- Add the soy sauce, rice wine vinegar and cashews and cook on high, allowing the liquid to reduce down to a sticky sauce.
- Serve hot, topped with sesame seeds and a drizzle of sesame oil.

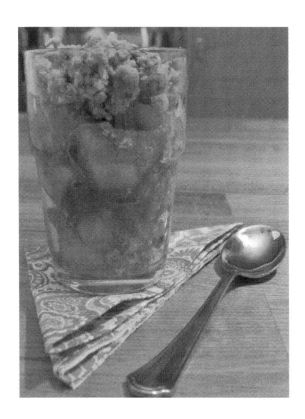

APPLE CRUMBLE

Ingredients:
2 Apples, peeled, cored and diced
2 tablespoons sugar free syrup – any flavour
¼ teaspoon cinnamon
Topping: High protein crumble mix – see recipe

METHOD
- Preheat oven 400F/200C/180c Fan/Gas 6
- Heat the apples, syrup and cinnamon in a pan until the apples are soft
- Spoon into 6 ramekins or similar
- Top with crumble mix

- Bake in the oven for 15 to 20 minutes or until topping is golden brown
- Serve warm

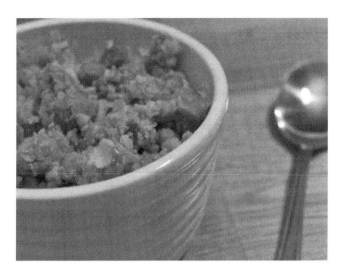

HIGH PROTEIN CRUMBLE MIX

Ingredients:
3 ½ tablespoons oats
3 ½ tablespoons oatmeal
3 ½ tablespoons protein powder – any flavour
3 ½ tablespoons chopped nuts – any
1 tablespoon peanut butter
1 tablespoon soft butter
1 tablespoon sugar free syrup – any flavour

METHOD
- Preheat oven 400F/200C/180c Fan/Gas 6
- Mix all of the ingredients in a bowl

- Line a flat baking tray with foil and spread the crumb mix over it
- Pop into the oven for approx. 10 minutes then remove and cool
- Use as a topping to desserts or as a base for Greek yoghurt topped with fresh soft fruit.

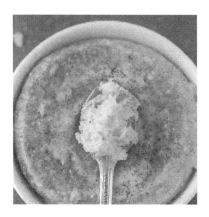

HIGH PROTEIN CINNAMON MUG CAKE

Ingredients:
1 scoop vanilla protein powder (32-34 grams)
1/2 tsp baking powder
1 tbsp coconut flour
1/2 tsp cinnamon
1 tbsp granulated sweetener of choice
1 large egg
1/4 cup milk of choice
1/4 tsp vanilla extract
1 tsp granulated sweetener of choice
1/2 tsp cinnamon
FOR THE GLAZE
1 tbsp coconut butter, melted
1/2 tsp milk of choice

A pinch of cinnamon

METHOD
- Grease a microwave safe bowl with cooking spray
- Add protein powder, baking powder, coconut flour, cinnamon, sweetener of choice and mix well
- Add the egg and mix into the dry mixture
- Add the milk and vanilla extract - If the batter is too crumbly continue adding milk until you have a very thick batter
- Mix the granulated sweetener and extra cinnamon and swirl over the top
- Microwave for 60 seconds, or until just cooked in the centre
- Top with glaze and serve

POUCH PORTIONS MEAL PLANNER: Weeks 1 to 3 – Liquids Only   1 TBSP per PP in Wk1   1 to 2 TBSP per PP in Wks 2&3

MEAL	DATE	Breakfast	Mid Morning	Lunch	Mid Afternoon	Dinner	Supper
Monday							
Tuesday							
Wednesday							
Thursday							
Friday							
Saturday							
Sunday							

Sip min of 1.5 ltr (3 pints) fluids per day – Eat 4 to 6 Pouch Portions per day - Check your weight twice a week

POUCH PORTIONS MEAL PLANNER: Weeks 4 to 6 – Puree Foods   ¼ Cup (or 4 TBSP) per PP

MEAL	DATE	Breakfast	Mid Morning	Lunch	Mid Afternoon	Dinner	Supper
Monday							
Tuesday							
Wednesday							
Thursday							
Friday							
Saturday							
Sunday							

Sip min of 1.5 ltr (3 pints) fluids per day – Eat 4 to 6 Pouch Portions per day - Check your weight twice a week

POUCH PORTIONS MEAL PLANNER: Weeks 7 to 9 – Soft Foods   ½ to 1 Cup(or 8 to 16 TBSP) per PP

MEAL	DATE	Breakfast	Mid Morning	Lunch	Mid Afternoon	Dinner	Supper
Monday							
Tuesday							
Wednesday							
Thursday							
Friday							
Saturday							
Sunday							

Sip min of 1.5 ltr (3 pints) fluids per day – Eat 3 Pouch Portions & 1 or 2 snacks – weight in once a week now

POUCH PORTIONS MEAL PLANNER: Weeks 10 & FOR LIFE 1 to 1 ½ cups (or 16 to 24 TBSP) per PP maximum

MEAL	DATE	Breakfast	Mid Morning	Lunch	Mid Afternoon	Dinner	Supper
Monday							
Tuesday							
Wednesday							
Thursday							
Friday							
Saturday							
Sunday							

Sip min of 1.5 ltr (3 pints) fluids per day – Eat 3 Pouch Portions & 1 or 2 snacks – weight in once a week now

Conversion Tables

Centigrade	Fahrenheit	Gas Mark	Descriptive	=	Fan Oven equiv. °C
110°	225°	¼	Very slow/Very low	=	90°
120°	250°	½	Very slow/Very low	=	100°
140°	275°	1	Slow/Low	=	120°
150°	300°	2	Slow/Low	=	130°
160°	325°	3	Moderately slow/Warm	=	140°
180°	350°	4	Moderate/Medium	=	160°
190°	375°	5	Moderate/Moderately hot	=	170°
200°	400°	6	Moderately hot	=	180°
220°	425°	7	Hot	=	200°
230°	450°	8	Hot/Very hot	=	210°
250°	475°	9	Very hot	=	230°
260°	500°	10	Extremely hot	=	240°

Cup	Tbsp	Oz
1/4	4	2
1/2	8	4
3/4	12	6
1	16	8
1.5	24	12
2	32	16

Afterward

Dear Pouch Portions, (PP) reader,

It's now 2019, and I've reached the 3rd year anniversary of my gastric bypass, and life is good.

It has taken me a long time to publish this book, but it's finally out there.

It feels like I've given birth!

You may recall me mentioning that I'd given my blender to my sister who was having surgery too? Well now "both" of my dear sisters have had the gastric bypass. They have done amazingly well, and I'm so proud of them.

Here's some before and after photos of the three of us.

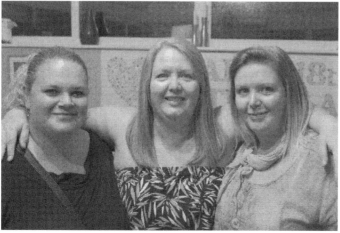

The three of us then . . .

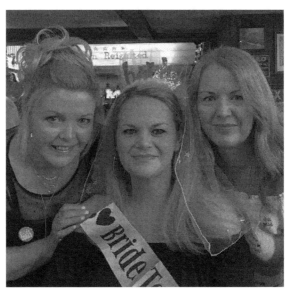
And the three of us now!

I'm still very mindful about what and how I eat, but not as much as I was during my first 2 years post op. And I haven't lost any more weight, in fact I've gained 8lbs.

"In the big scheme of thing that's not too bad" I hear you say.

But it's a slippery slope dear PP reader.

If you're not careful you can easily slip back into your old eating habits. Food is much easier to eat now, your Pouch Portions have gotten bigger, and that second glass of wine you steered clear of in the past is calling your name. One more won't hurt will it?

Before you know it your scales are screaming at you to get off, your clothes are tighter, and you're beating yourself up every time you eat or drink too much.

As I said at the beginning of this book, bariatric surgery is a tool. Not a magic wand.

You still have to put in the hard work, stick to the rules, exercise and keep those lifestyle changes going that you made at the start of your journey.

I'm currently working hard on getting back on track and getting rid of those pesky pounds. I've gone back on the LSD of 2shakes a day with a light protein dinner. And I've cut out alcohol completely, (which is a shame as I'm loving this gin revival that's going on at the moment).

I love food and drink as much as the next person, but I love being slim and healthy even more!

If we aren't mindful about what we put into our bodies, then why have the surgery in the first place?

Enjoy your bariatric journey. You won't regret it, and if my words have helped you in any way I'm happy.

I wish you love, joy and abundance in all you do dear PP reader.

Mandy x

Printed in Great
Britain
by Amazon